Paleo 30 Days of Thanks

Tasty Gluten-Free Gifts to Share with Friends

Lucy Fast

Just to say Thank You for Purchasing this Book I want to give you a gift 100% absolutely FREE

A Copy of My Special Report

"Paleo Pantry: The Beginner's Guide to What Should and Should NOT be in Your Paleo Kitchen"

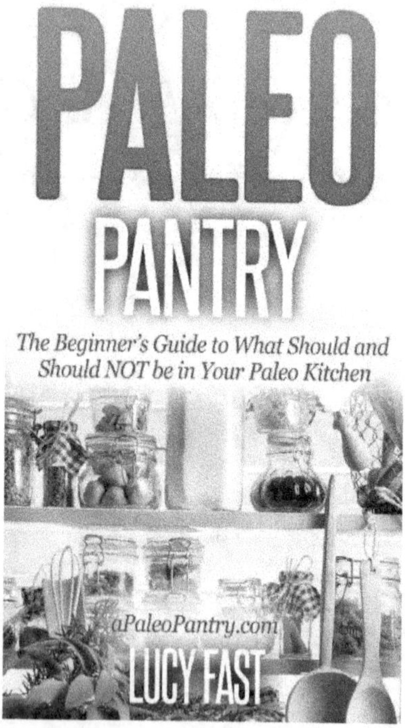

Go to www.aPaleoPantry.com to

Reserve your FREE copy

Disclaimer and Terms of Use: The Author and Publisher have strived to be as accurate and complete as possible in the creation of this book, notwithstanding the fact that they do not warrant or represent at any time that the contents within are accurate due to the rapidly changing nature of the Internet. While all attempts have been made to verify information provided in this publication, the Author and Publisher assume no responsibility for errors, omissions, or contrary interpretation of the subject matter herein. Any perceived slights of specific persons, peoples, or organizations are unintentional. In practical advice books, like anything else in life, there are no guarantees of income made or health benefits received. This book is not intended for use as a source of medical, legal, business, accounting or financial advice. All readers are advised to seek services of competent professionals in medical, legal, business, accounting, and finance matters.

Printed in the United States of America

Table of Contents

Introduction

Thanksgiving is the true kick-off to the holiday season, yet it tends to get overshadowed by the bigger winter holidays. Consumers in the United States are greeted with Halloween in August and Christmas in October. Our traditional November holiday gets lost in the woodwork. Even the following day (Black Friday) has tried to steal some of Thanksgiving's thunder.

Thankfully (no pun intended), we have started to restore some focus back on the holiday that celebrates gratitude. The 30 Days of Thanks movement that began several years ago takes social media by storm every year on the first day of November. This project involves stating one thing you are thankful for each day throughout the month of November.

In this book, we're taking the 30 Days of Thanks concept one step further. What better way to show gratitude for the folks that you value than by writing them a sweet note or card attached to a homemade gift, a token of your thanks? Better yet, they're all Paleo-friendly and gluten-free! You'll find:

- Make-ahead treats
- Jar mixes for the pantry
- Unique blends of salts, sugars, and spices
- Tips on writing genuine thank-you notes

What are you waiting for? Let's get thankin'!

Lucy

How To Thank-You

Sometimes it's hard to find the "just right" words to say to someone. The greeting card industry exists because of this truth! While a store-bought card with a pre-written message suffices for plenty of situations, there are times when you want to express a more personal note than the one already included in the card. If you struggle with writing (and most people do), here are some tips on how to compose a genuine and heartfelt thank-you note.

1. Write the way that you speak

There's a huge misconception out there that you have to write on some Shakespearian level of eloquence in order to communicate effectively. The myth buster is this: When writing a personal message, use the same tone of voice and words that you would use as if you were speaking directly to that person…because you are speaking directly to that person!

2. Be clear about what you are thanking the person for

Whether it's a gift you received or a small service they performed that meant the world to you, let the note's recipient know just what they did that you appreciate.

3. Explain why you appreciate the gift or service

If someone brought you a meal while you were sick, thank him or her for the meal, and go on to explain why it was so meaningful to you. Likewise, if somebody sent you a new set of knives as a wedding gift, let them know how this set is an instant upgrade from the old knives you were using and how it will make your life in the kitchen so much easier.

4. Keep it short

In order to thank somebody, you don't have to be over the top. You just have to be authentic.

The Daily Difference

When we consider what and who we are thankful for, our families and closest friends are typically at the top of the list: husbands, wives, parents, siblings, children, and BFFS get the headline.

Once we step aside from our nucleus of relationships, however, the list might seem a bit more challenging. It's not that you aren't thankful for anyone else, it's just that you are actually required to think a little more about your life, your circumstances, and the people in your world who act to make everything positive.

People like:

- Your teachers
- Your children's teachers
- The principal at their school
- Your mail carrier
- Your next-door neighbors
- Your handyman
- The teenager who mows your lawn
- Your favorite librarian
- Your favorite teller at the bank
- Your babysitter
- The crossing guard
- The receptionist or secretary at work who always jokes with you and makes sure your messages are delivered
- The IT guy or gal at work who fixes your dumb computer
- The custodian or janitor who always greets you with a smile or asks about your day

- The mechanic who is always straight with you about your vehicle
- The person at your church who gives a lot of their time to a program you are involved with
- The barista or bartender who goes ahead and makes your favorite drink when they see you walk through the door
- The couple you talk to when you take your daily walk through the neighborhood
- The farmer at the farmer's market who throws in a freebie for you

These are just a few of the people in your neighborhood and your daily world who do things you surely appreciate. How many more can you come up with for these 30 Days of Thanks?

Iced Winter Tea

Ingredients:

3 c. water
1 large orange, cut into thin slices
1 three-inch cinnamon stick, cut in half
6 whole cloves
5 decaffeinated black tea bags
1 1/2 c. freshly squeezed orange juice
1 1/2 c. pomegranate juice
3 T. coconut sugar
1 glass pitcher

***Directions*:**

1. Combine first four ingredients in a medium pan over high heat.
2. Remove from stove once mixture begins to boil.
3. Add tea bags, and place lid on top of pot.
4. Allow mixture to stand for 10 minutes.
5. Remove bags, and discard.
6. Strain mixture, and remove oranges and whole spices.
7. In a glass pitcher, combine tea with juices and sugar until dissolved.
8. Cover and chill for at least five hours.
9. To give as a gift, tie a ribbon around the pitcher handle with instructions to stir and serve over ice.

Makes 7 cups (7 1-cup servings)

Fall Granola

Ingredients:

¼ c. pure Maple syrup
2 T. coconut oil
2 T. grass-fed butter
1 t. vanilla extract
1 c. pepitas
1 c. raw walnuts
1 c. raw cashews
2 c. finely shredded coconut
½ c. dried apples, chopped
½ c. dried cherries
½ c. dried cranberries

Directions:

1. Preheat oven to 350°F
2. In a 13x9 inch pan, combine syrup, oil, and butter. Melt in oven (about 5 minutes).
3. Add vanilla, pepitas, walnuts, and cashews. Stir to coat.
4. Bake for 25-30 minutes, stirring every 7-8 minutes.
5. Turn off the oven, and stir in coconut, baking for an additional 5 minutes.
6. Remove from oven, cool completely.
7. Stir in dried fruit.

Makes 6 (1-cup) serving

Lavender Vanilla Coconut Sugar

Ingredients:

2 lbs. coconut sugar
3 tsp. dried lavender
1 vanilla bean

Directions:

1. In a large bowl, mix the sugar and lavender.
2. Scrape out the vanilla bean seeds, mix in with sugar and lavender.
3. Bury the vanilla bean "stick" into the sugar.
4. Let sit for 10 days in an airtight container.

Makes enough to fill 8-10 small jars for gift giving

Brownie Mix

Ingredients:

1 c. coconut sugar
½ c. almond flour
1/3 c. unsweetened cocoa
¼ tsp. fine sea salt
¼ tsp. baking soda
¼ tsp. cream of tartar

Directions:

1. Combine all dry ingredients in a large bowl, whisking together.
2. Store in an airtight container until ready to use.
3. When ready to use, add 2 eggs, ½ c. coconut oil, and 1 tsp. of vanilla, baking for 25 minutes at 350°F.

Makes 1 mix (1 mix = 1 pan of brownies)

Paleo Ranch Mix

Ingredients:

3 tsp. dried dill
3 tsp. garlic powder
3 tsp. onion powder
3 tsp. dried parsley
1 tsp. dried thyme
2 ¾ tsp. black pepper
4 tsp. fine sea salt

Directions:

1. Combine all ingredients in a small bowl, whisking together.

Makes ½ c. of ranch mix

Apple Pie Snack Mix

Ingredients:

1 c. coconut flakes
1 c. dried apples, chopped
1 c. golden raisins
1 c. walnuts
1 T. coconut oil
¼ tsp. vanilla extract
¼ tsp. cinnamon
¼ tsp. ginger
¼ tsp. cloves
¼ tsp. fine sea salt

***Directions*:**

1. Pre-heat a large skillet over medium-high heat.
2. Add coconut flakes, and stir constantly for 2-3 minutes or until toasted. Remove from heat.
3. In a medium bowl, mix coconut with apples and raisins, set aside.
4. In the same skillet, melt oil over medium heat. Add walnuts, and stir to coat.
5. Add extract and seasonings, stirring to glaze (about 2-3 minutes). Remove from heat and cool.
6. Stir glazed walnuts into apple mixture.

Makes 8 (1/2 cup) servings.

Gingerbread Spice Mix

Ingredients:

¼ c. ground cinnamon
¼ c. ground ginger
¼ c. ground cloves
¼ c. ground allspice
3 tsp. black pepper

***Directions*:**

1. Mix together in a small bowl and store in an airtight container.

Bacon Salt

Ingredients:

1 lb. bacon, cooked, and slightly cooled
1 ½ T. Celtic sea salt
2 tsp. black pepper

Directions:

1. Place all ingredients in a food processor and process until very fine. Store in an airtight container and refrigerate.

Mulling Spices

Ingredients:

12 pieces of cheesecloth cut into 6-inch circles
5 half-inch cinnamon sticks
5 star anise
10 cardamom pods
20 black peppercorns
1 ¼ tsp. whole cloves
Twine

Directions:

1. Layer 2 pieces of cheesecloth together.
2. In the center, place ½ a cinnamon stick, a star anise, 2 pods of cardamom, 5 peppercorns, and ¼ tsp. cloves.
3. Tie with twine.
4. Repeat until you have 5 bags of mulling spices.
5. Store in a decorative tin or other airtight container.

Makes 5 bags of mulling spices.

Spiced Apple Tea Mix

Ingredients:

2 T. loose decaffeinated green tea or white green tea
2 T. crystallized ginger, chopped
1 tsp. whole allspice
1 tsp. whole cloves
6 slices of dried apple slices
6 3-inch cinnamon sticks
6 paper tea bags or tea filters
Kitchen string

Directions:

1. In a small bowl, thoroughly combine all ingredients except for apples and cinnamon.
2. Evenly scoop tea mixture into tea bags.
3. Place 1 apple slice in each tea bag.
4. Using kitchen string, tie a cinnamon stick to the tops of tea bags or filters.
5. Give in a clear, glass, decorative container or in individual teacups.
6. Attach directions: Pour 8 ounces hot water over tea bag and let steep for 3 to 5 minutes. Remove and discard tea bag.

Makes 6 bags of tea, which will brew 6 cups of tea

Spicy Nuts

Ingredients:

2 c. pecan halves
2 c. walnut halve
4 T. pure maple syrup
2½ T. coconut oil
4 T. coconut sugar
2 T. ground ancho chili powder

Directions:

1. Preheat oven to 250 degrees and line a 13x9x2-inch baking pan with foil.
2. In a medium bowl, stir together nuts, syrup, and oil until nuts are coated.
3. Stir in sugar and chili powder.
4. Spread mixture on prepared pan, pressing as you go to make sure the mixture is even.
5. Bake for 45 minutes, stirring every 15 minutes.
6. Spread on a large, heatproof surface to cool.
7. Store in airtight container at room temperature for 2 weeks or freeze for up to 1 month.

Makes 2-1/2 cups (1 serving = ¾ cup)

Spiced Dry Rub

Ingredients:

6 T. dried chili flakes
6 T. dried thyme
4 T. dried rosemary
2 T. rubbed sage
4 bay leaves, crushed
2 tsp. celery salt
4 tsp. garlic powder
4 T. peppercorns

Directions:

1. Whisk together all the ingredients in a small bowl.
2. Store in an airtight container or a pepper grinder.

Makes 1 c. of spice mix.

Tropical Lime & Ginger Salt

Ingredients:

6 limes, zested
3 tsp. ground ginger
1 c. Celtic fine sea salt

Directions:

1. Spread lime zest on a cookie sheet lined with wax paper, and let air-dry overnight.
2. The next day, combine zest with ginger and salt in a small bowl. Store in an airtight jar.

Makes 1 cup of salt.

Euro Herbes de Provence Salt

Ingredients:

½ c. herbes de Provence
6 T. dried lavender
¾ c. fine sea salt

Directions:

1. In a spice grinder or food processor, pulse herbes and lavender until coarsely ground.
2. In a small bowl, whisk together herbes mixture with salt. Store in an airtight jar.

Makes 1 cup of salt

Salted Caramel Sauce

Ingredients:

½ c. full-fat coconut milk or coconut cream
1 c. coconut sugar
1/3 c. water
½ c. grass-fed butter
¼ tsp. Vanilla
¼ tsp. flaky sea salt

Directions:

1. Chill coconut milk or cream for 8 hours or overnight.
2. In a heavy saucepan over medium-high heat, combine sugar and water. Refrain from stirring, and allow to heat until the sugar begins to melt and brown.
3. Tilt the pan around so that the sugar browns evenly, cooking for 5-7 minutes or until golden.
4. Remove from heat, and add butter. Stir until butter melts.
5. Pour in coconut milk, vanilla, and salt, and stir.
6. Cool completely, and refrigerate in an airtight container for 2 weeks.

Makes 1 cup of sauce.

Cherry Ginger Pancakes

Ingredients:

1 T. whey powder
¼ c. sugar
3 tsp. baking soda
1 tsp. cream of tartar
½ tsp. fine sea salt
¾ tsp. ground ginger
32-oz. container or 1 qt. glass jar
2 c. almond flour
¾ c. dried cherries
½ c. almond flour or cornmeal
2 T. finely chopped crystallized ginger

***Directions*:**

1. Combine first six ingredients together in a medium bowl.
2. In your container or jar, layer the following ingredients in order from bottom to top: flour, dried cherries, flour or cornmeal, and chopped ginger.
3. Store the layered jar of pancake ingredients at room temperature up to 1 month.
4. To make pancakes, whisk 1 egg, ¾ c. water, and 2 T. coconut oil with dry ingredients until combined. Let rest for five minutes.

Makes 10 to 12 standard-size pancakes

Cranberry Chutney

Ingredients:

1¼ c. coconut sugar
½ c. freshly squeezed orange juice
3 c. fresh cranberries
1 c. peeled, cored and chopped apples
1 c. golden raisins
¼ c. coconut sugar
1 T. molasses
2 tsp. minced fresh ginger

Directions:

1. Combine granulated sugar and orange juice in a large saucepan.
2. Cook and stir over medium-high heat until sugar is dissolved. Then, without stirring, bring the mixture to a boil.
3. Stir in all remaining ingredients, and bring to a boil once again.
4. Reduce heat to medium, and simmer for 5 minutes, or until mixture is thicker and berries have begun to burst.
5. Remove from heat and let cool.
6. Refrigerate in an airtight container for up to a week.

Makes 3½ cups chutney.

Sweet Chili Jam

Ingredients:

8 red bell peppers, chopped
10 red chilies, chopped
3-inch piece of ginger, peeled and chopped
8 garlic cloves, peeled
3½ c. cherry tomatoes
3¾ c. coconut sugar
4 T. molases
2 c. red wine vinegar

***Directions*:**

1. Place peppers, ginger, and chilies in a food processor. Pulse until chopped fine.
2. Add mixture to heavy saucepan.
3. Add all remaining ingredients, and bring to a boil.
4. Skim surface scum, lower heat to a simmer, and cook for 1 hour, stirring occasionally.
5. When the jam becomes sticky, cook for an additional 10-15 minutes, and stir frequently.
6. Once the jam is thick and bubbly, remove from heat, and cool for 10-15 minutes before transferring the jam to airtight jars that have been sterilized.

Makes 4 small jars of jam

Whole Grain Honey Mustard

Ingredients:

2 c. Yellow mustard seeds
1 c. Brown mustard seeds
1 ¼ c. champagne vinegar
1 clove of garlic
1 tsp. crushed red pepper
1 6-inch cinnamon stick
1/3 c. honey
1 fine sea salt

Directions:

1. In a bowl, mix together first six ingredients. Cover and set aside for one full day (24 hour period).
2. Discard cinnamon stick, and add honey, stirring well to combine.
3. Blend 2¼ cups of mixture in a food processor until finely pureed and ground.
4. Add remaining mixture and sea salt, and stir.
5. Spoon into sterilized jars.

Makes 3 cups mustard.

Rosemary & Mint Honey

Ingredients:

8 c. honey
10 fresh rosemary sprigs

Directions:

1. In a medium saucepan over low heat, cook honey, 6 sprigs rosemary, and 3 mint leaves just until honey begins to bubble around the edges.
2. Remove from heat.
3. Allow mixture to rest for 20 minutes.
4. Remove all leaves from mixture.
3. Divide honey into clean glass jars. Cool completely. Place unused rosemary springs in each jar. Tighten to seal.

Makes 4 cups of honey.

Golden Autumn Granola

Ingredients:

5 c. mixed raw nuts
1 c. pepitas
1 c. dried cranberries
1 c. chopped dried apricots
1 c. golden raisins
1 c. coconut sugar
2 T. molasses
1 tsp. ground cinnamon
½ tsp. sea salt
1½ stick grass-fed butter
1/2 c. honey

Directions:

1. Preheat oven to 350°F. Line a baking sheet with parchment paper, and set aside.
2. In a large bowl, combine all ingredients except butter and honey. Set aside.
3. In the meantime, melt butter in a small saucepan over medium heat.
4. Stir in honey.
5. Pour honey mixture over nut mixture, and stir until well coated.
6. Bake for 35-40 minutes until nuts are toasted and sugars melt.
7. Cool and transfer to an airtight container.

Makes 10 cups granola.

Choco-candy cane nibbles

Ingredients:

1 1/3 c. dates, pitted (soaked in boiling water for at least 10 minutes)
1 1/3 c. unsweetened shredded coconut
4 T. cacao powder
½ c. coconut oil
4-6 drops of pure peppermint oil

Directions:

1. Soak dates in boiling water for 10-15 minutes or until plump. Drain and set aside.
2. Place coconut and cacao in food processor. Process until finely ground.
3. With the processor still on, add dates and oils, and process until smooth and paste-like.
4. Using a rubber spatula, scrape mixture into a large mixing bowl, and stir.
5. Roll ¼ c. portions of mixture into small balls. Set on a baking sheet.
6. Chill for half an hour, and store in an airtight container, refrigerated, for up to 10 days.

Makes 24 balls.

Pumpkin Chocolate Chip Cookie Mix

* You can go ahead and make the cookies, or gift the mix with instructions—your call!

Ingredients:

¼ c. coconut sugar
1 T. cream of tartar
2 ½ tsp. baking soda
1 T. pumpkin pie spice
½ tsp. baking soda
1/8 tsp. fine Celtic sea salt
½ c. dark chocolate chips

Add on baking day:

⅔ c. canned pumpkin
½ c. almond butter
1 egg, beaten
1 ½ tsp. pure vanilla extract

Directions:

1. Add all ingredients in bowl, and mix well until combined. Store in an airtight container with instructions for what to add on baking day.
2. On baking day, mix in a large bowl the wet ingredients with the dry.
3. Drop or roll tablespoons of batter onto a baking sheet lined with parchment paper.
4. Baking for 15-18 minutes at 350 degrees until golden.

Makes 16 cookies

Southern Slow-Cooked Apple Pumpkin Butter

Ingredients:

5 lbs. cooking apples, unpeeled, cored, and diced
¼ c. unsweetened apple cider
1 ¼ c. coconut sugar, divided
2 T. cinnamon, divided
1 15-oz can canned pumpkin
1 tsp. ground cloves
1 tsp. freshly grated nutmeg
1 tsp. ground ginger
1 lemon, juiced
1/8 tsp. fine sea salt

Directions:

1. In a slow cooker, stir together apples, juice/cider, ½ c. coconut sugar, and 1 T. cinnamon. Cook on LOW for 8-9 hours or until apples are tender.
2. Remove apple mixture from crock, and let cool.
3. Pour half of apple mixture into a food processor, and puree until completely smooth. Remove and pour into a large bowl. Process the remaining mixture.
4. Return apple mixture to slow cooker along with all remaining ingredients, stirring well to combine.
5. Cook on HIGH for 6-8 hours until dark in color and slightly reduced.
6. Pour into glass jars and refrigerate for 2 weeks, or freeze for half a year.

Makes 3½ pints

Homemade Peppermint Extract

Ingredients:

1 large bunch peppermint, or ½ c. peppermint leaves, packed
1½ c. vodka

***Directions*:**

1. Rinse mint leaves in a strainer.
2. Using your hands, squeeze the leaves of extra moisture.
3. Pour vodka over mint to cover leaves.
4. Place entire mixture in a jar, and store in a cool, dark place for 3-4 weeks.
5. Strain leaves, and use extract.

Makes 1 pint of extract.

Note - You can also make Vanilla or Cinnamon extract just as easily. Simply replace the mint in the recipe above with one split whole vanilla bean or 2-3 cinnamon sticks.

Georgia Brittle

Ingredients:

½ c. pecans
½ c. raw honey
½ c. pure maple syrup
½ c. coconut oil, divided
¼ c. almond butter
½ c. Coconut cream
2 tsp. cinnamon
1 tsp. vanilla extract
1/8 tsp. fine sea salt

Directions:

1. Preheat a medium saucepan over a medium flame, and line an 8x8 baking dish with parchment paper.
2. Melt 1 T. coconut oil.
3. Add pecans, stirring to coat, cooking until slightly browned.
4. Immediately add honey and syrup, stirring to coat and until slightly thickened.
5. Add and mix together almond butter, remaining coconut oil, and coconut cream.
6. Add all remaining ingredients, stirring to combine.
7. Set heat on low, simmering for a few minutes until just slightly thickened.
8. Spoon mixture into baking dish, making sure it is even.

9. Freeze for 1-2 hours.
10. Remove from freezer, and cut into pieces. Store in a freezer-safe container.

Makes 4 servings.

Chocolate Cashew Butter

Ingredients:

1 ¼ c. unsalted cashews
1 tsp. coconut oil, melted
2 oz. dark chocolate, melted
1/8 tsp. fine sea salt

Directions:

1. Process cashews in food processor until smooth (7-8 minutes), scraping as needed.
2. Add oil and chocolate slowly through the processor stream.
3. Add salt.
4. Store in air-tight container in the refrigerator.

Makes ½ cup butter.

Roasted Garlic Oil

Ingredients:

3 large heads garlic
3 cups olive oil

Directions:

1. Preheat the oven to 300°F.
2. Cut garlic in half horizontally, and place cut-side down in an ovenproof casserole.
3. Pour oil over garlic, and bake for 1 hour or until tender.
4. Pour oil into strainer placed over a bowl. Let cool. Store in an airtight container.

Makes 2½ c. garlic oil

White Toasted Almond Bark

Ingredients:

1 cup whole raw almonds
20 oz. white chocolate, chopped
1-2 T. fine Celtic sea salt

Directions:

1. Preheat oven to 350°F.
2. Spread almonds onto a baking sheet, and bake for 20 minutes, stirring occasionally. Let cool.
3. In the meantime, prepare a second baking sheet lined with parchment paper.
4. Melt chocolate in a double boiler, stirring constantly until smooth.
5. Add almonds to chocolate, and stir until coated.
6. Spread almond mixture onto lined baking sheet, and sprinkle evenly with sea salt.
7. Refrigerate for an hour.
8. Remove from refrigerator, and break into pieces.

Makes 2 cups almond bark.

Tropical Banana Bread

Ingredients:

Coconut oil spray
½ c. coconut flour
2 tsp. baking soda
1 tsp. cream of tartar
1/8 tsp. Sea salt
1 tsp. Vanilla
4 T. coconut oil
½ c. almond butter
4 eggs
1½ c. mashed bananas
1 c. crushed pineapple, drained well
1/3 c. unsweetened shredded coconut

Directions:

1. Preheat your oven to 350° F. Spray 2 loaf pans with coconut oil spray and set aside.
2. Whisk together dry ingredients in a large bowl. Set aside.
3. In another bowl, mix together wet ingredients.
4. Add wet to dry, and mix well.
5. Bake for 45-50 minutes or until a toothpick inserted into breads comes out clean.

Makes 2 loaves

Conclusion

For all that others do for us, it's the least we can do to show our appreciation. We hope you've found our recipes easy, quick, nutritious, and delicious! Why not set a day aside during which you make gifts for everyone on your thirty days of thanks list? Don't forget to save some for yourself. The mixes and salts last in the pantry, and the chutneys and jams are great to have on hand during the busy holiday season!

Lucy Fast

Check out Lucy's other books!!

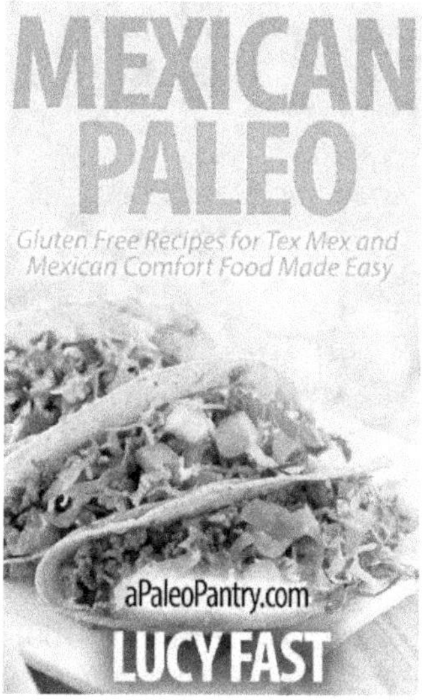

http://www.amazon.com/dp/B00J1UOLMI

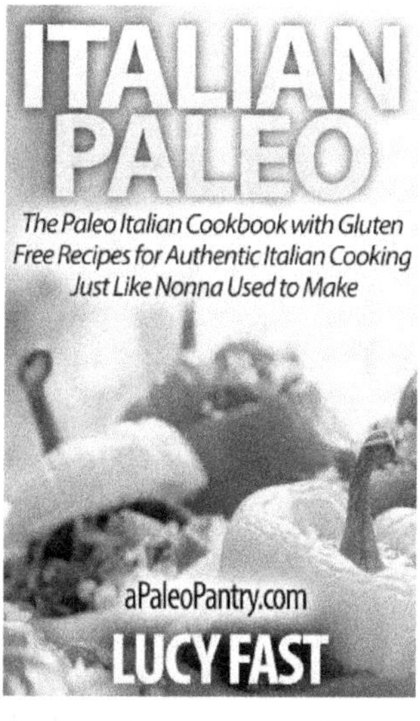

http://www.amazon.com/dp/B00J1TU18C

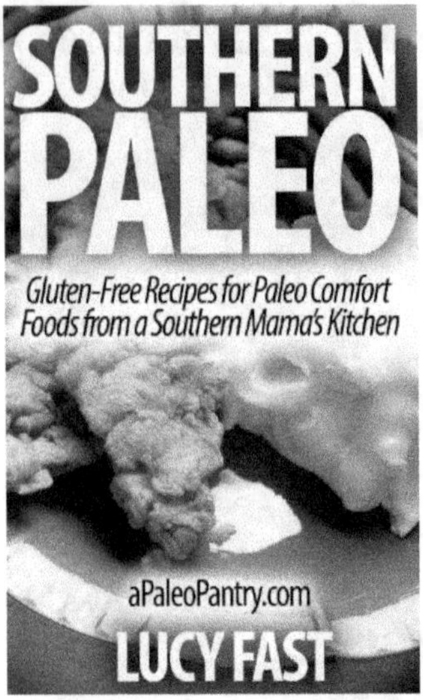

http://www.amazon.com/dp/B00HYKJCZ8

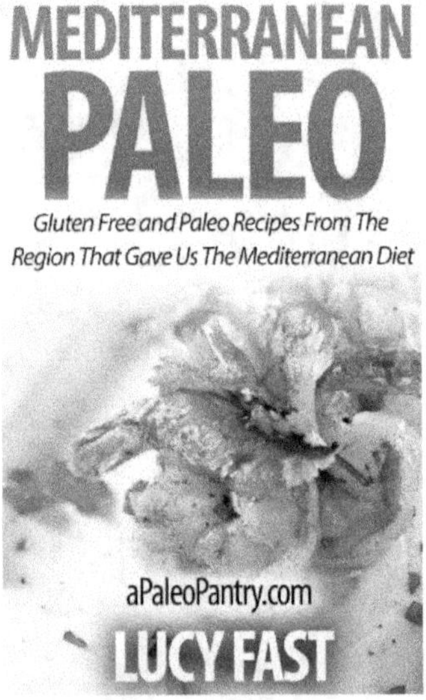

http://www.amazon.com/dp/B00JV4FNXU

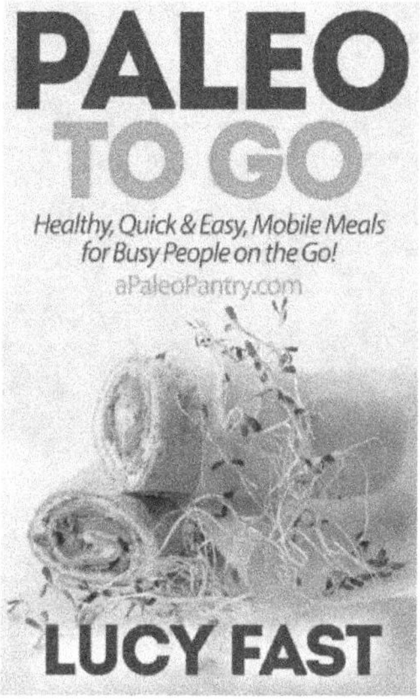

http://www.amazon.com/dp/B00HH1GBLC

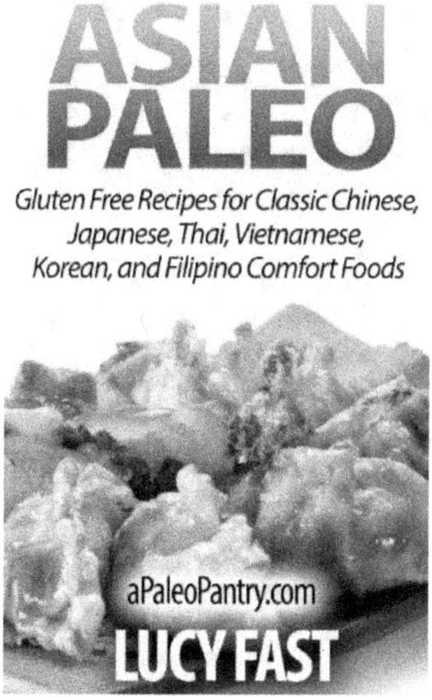

http://www.amazon.com/dp/B00JOS53H4

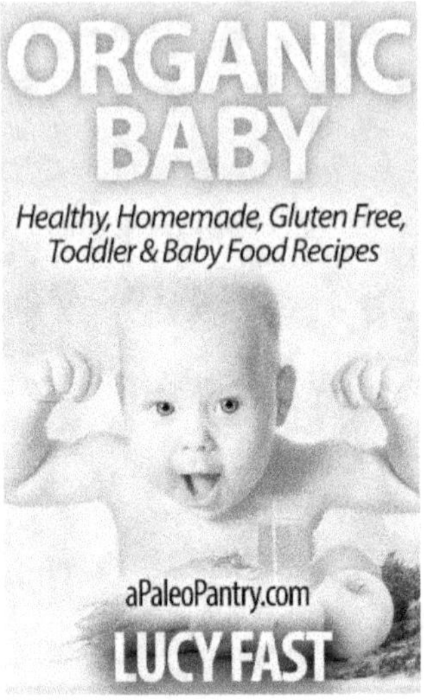

http://www.amazon.com/dp/B00I4MDXVO

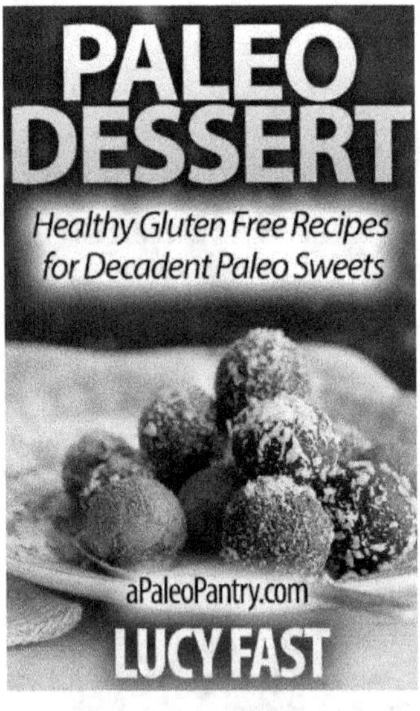

http://www.amazon.com/dp/B00JOWF758

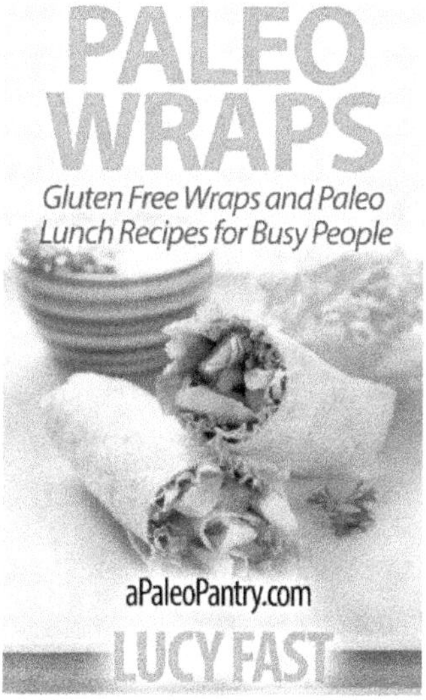

http://www.amazon.com/dp/B00IIHKA84

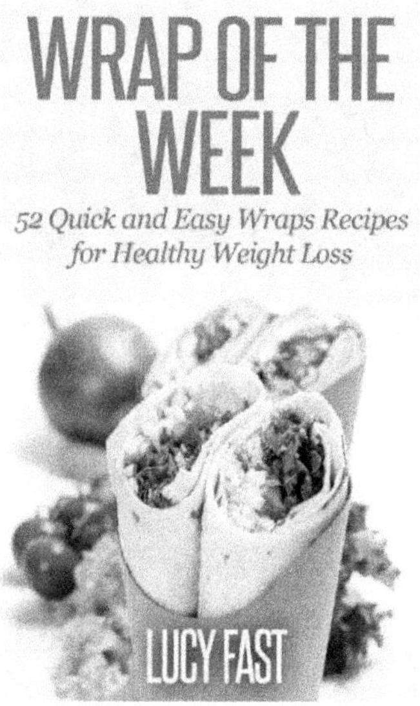

http://www.amazon.com/dp/B00KBA9HNK

www.ingramcontent.com/pod-product-compliance
Lightning Source LLC
Chambersburg PA
CBHW060651290526
45793CB00001B/493
9781505228427